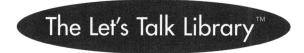
The Let's Talk Library™

Let's Talk About Being Overweight

Melanie Apel Gordon

The Rosen Publishing Group's
PowerKids Press™
New York

Dedicated to Jennifer Costin Thomas and a friendship to last a lifetime. 1973–forever.
Love, Melanie

Published in 2000 by The Rosen Publishing Group, Inc.
29 East 21st Street, New York, NY 10010

First Edition

Book Design: Erin McKenna

Photo Credits and Photo Illustrations: pp. 4, 7, 8, 19, 20 by Debra Marcus Brown; p. 11 © Hal Kern/International Stock; pp. 12, 16 © Skjold Photographs; p. 15 © Lou Manna/International Stock.

Gordon, Melanie Apel.
    Let's talk about being overweight / by Melanie Apel Gordon.
        p.   cm.— (The Let's talk library)
    Includes index.
    Summary: Discusses the unhealthy aspects of being overweight, the relationship between weight and a program of diet and exercise, and ways to stay physically fit.
    ISBN 0-8239-5413-7 (lib. bdg.)
    1. Obesity—Juvenile literature. [1. Obesity. 2. Weight control.] I. Title. II. Series.
RC628.G675 1998
616.3'98—dc21   98-45439
                                                                                          CIP
                                                                                          AC

Manufactured in the United States of America

Contents

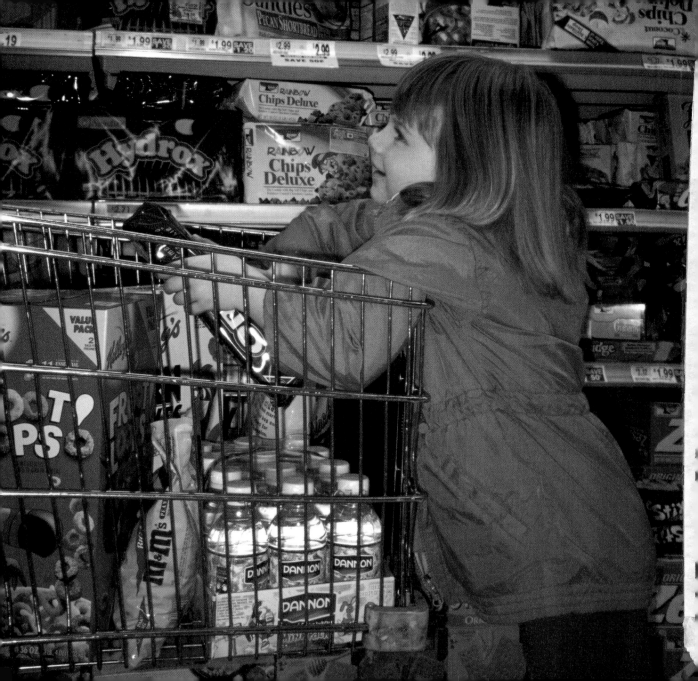

Jill

Jill and her mother are at the supermarket. Jill keeps putting cookies and junk food into the shopping cart. Jill's mother is worried. Jill eats lots of junk food and hardly ever eats vegetables. Jill has gained a lot of weight recently. "Jill, you're not healthy," her mom says. "Maybe we should buy more healthful food and less junk food."

◀ *Even though junk food tastes good, it's not very good for your body.*

Being Overweight

About 7 million children and one in every three adults in the United States are **overweight**. Being overweight means that you weigh more than is healthy for your age and height. This is most often because there is too much fat in your body. It's okay to weigh more than your friends. That just means that your body is different from theirs. However, if your weight makes it hard for you to **exercise** or do things that you want to do, then you may not be as healthy as you could be.

Being overweight can make kids feel bad about themselves. ▶

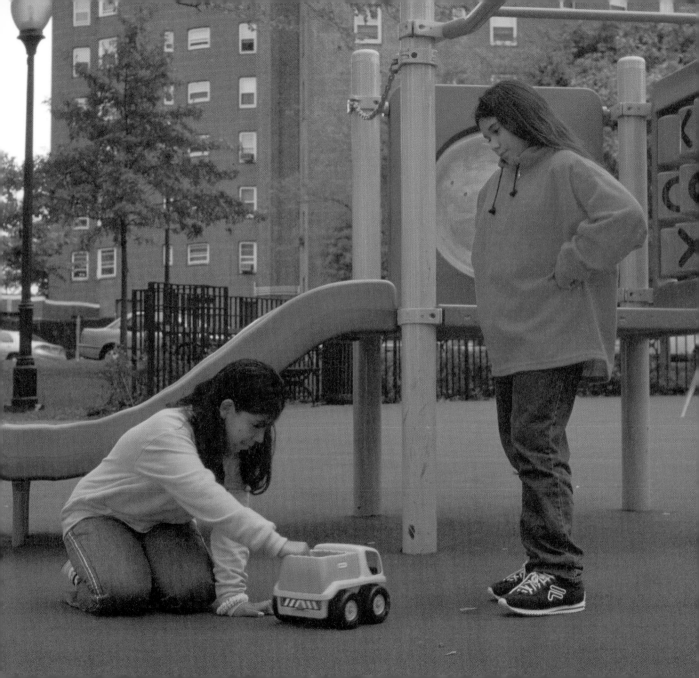

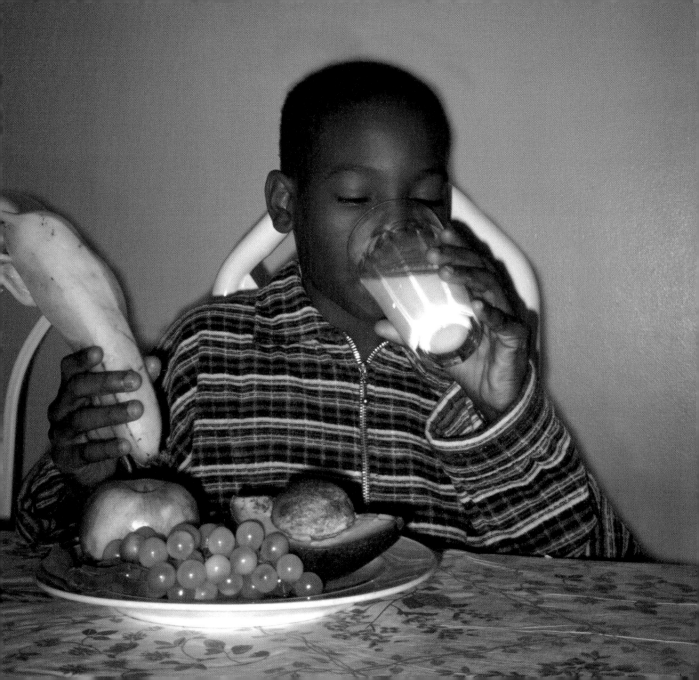

How Did I Gain Weight?

Our bodies use the food we eat as **fuel**. Some foods are better fuel than others. Vegetables, lean meats, and grains are the best fuel. Sugars and fats aren't very good fuel. When we eat, our bodies use the best fuel first. Anything that is left gets stored as fat. If we exercise a lot, that fat gets used up. But if we don't exercise, that fat stays on our bodies. Most people are overweight because they eat too much fatty food and they do not exercise enough.

◀ *Eating fresh fruits and vegetables is a good way to get nutrients and stay healthy.*

Growing

When you were a baby you probably had a lot of fat in your body. That's okay. You were healthy. As you grow and your body changes, you lose the extra fat that your body no longer needs. Some fat will stay on your body so that you can be healthy. But it is not healthy for too much fat to stay on your body. Eating well and being active helps you keep the right amount of fat in your body.

Babies need more fat in their bodies than older kids do. ▶

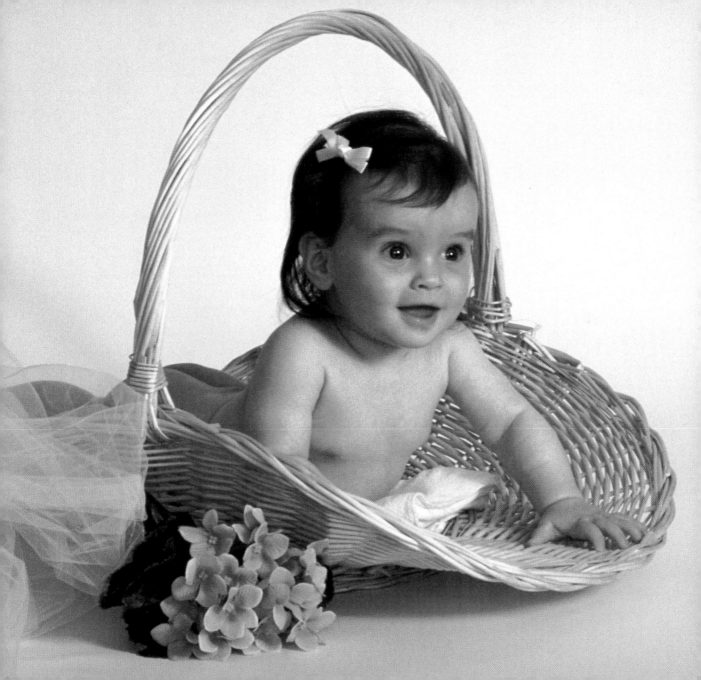

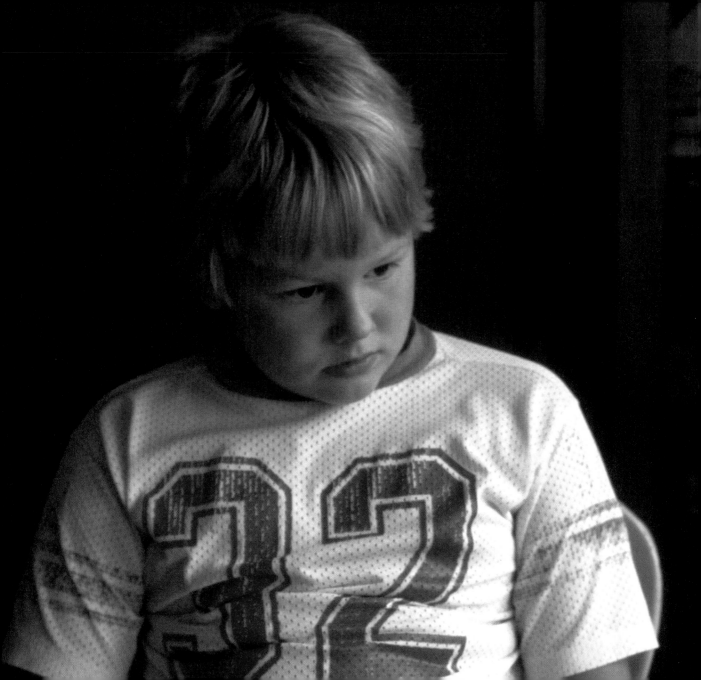

It's a Problem

Being overweight makes it hard for your body to work **efficiently**. If you are overweight you may get tired and out of breath from walking or climbing stairs. You may also have a hard time running or playing sports. It takes a lot of **energy** to run around and be active when you are overweight. If it's hard for you be active, then you may choose NOT to be active. However, being active is very important for growing kids.

◀ *When kids aren't active, they get tired easily. Their bodies are less healthy than they could be.*

The Food You Eat

If you are overweight, you are probably not eating a **well-balanced diet**. Your diet is the food you eat. Your growing body needs healthful foods. Fruits, vegetables, meats, breads, and small amounts of fatty foods such as cheese and peanut butter make a good diet. It's even okay to eat some junk food. However, eating only a little bit of junk food is better for you and your body. If you eat mostly healthful food and stay active, your body will be healthier.

*Just because you should eat in a healthful way doesn't ▶
mean you can't eat foods you like. Pizza is healthful.*

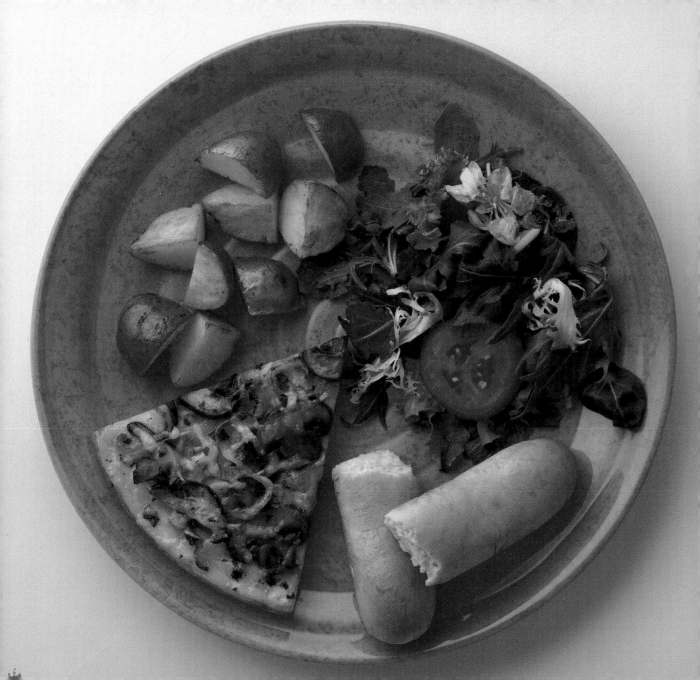

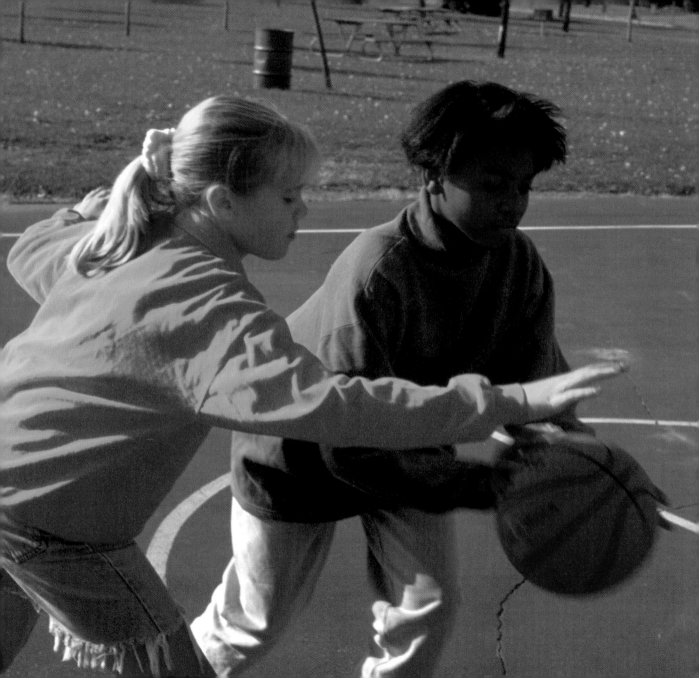

Being Active Is Fun

One of the best ways to stay healthy is to be active. Playing sports, running around outdoors, dancing, and skating are all fun ways to be active. This exercise helps your body build strong bones and muscles, which helps keep you from being overweight. If you are already overweight, you might need to be a little more active. Pick a fun activity. It will feel good to use your body. Plus, the better you get at that activity, the better you will feel about yourself.

◀ *Playing a game with your friends is a fun way to exercise.*

Kids Have the Power!

Did you know that you have the power to have a healthy body? Well, you do. If you watch TV, you may see lots of commercials for junk food. But you don't have to eat that stuff. Decide for yourself what to eat. You also have the power to say "no" to watching TV, and "yes" to being active. For a healthier body, try to spend a little less time in front of the TV or playing video games, and spend a little more time outdoors.

It's okay to play video games for a little while. Just try to spend some time each day being active. ▶

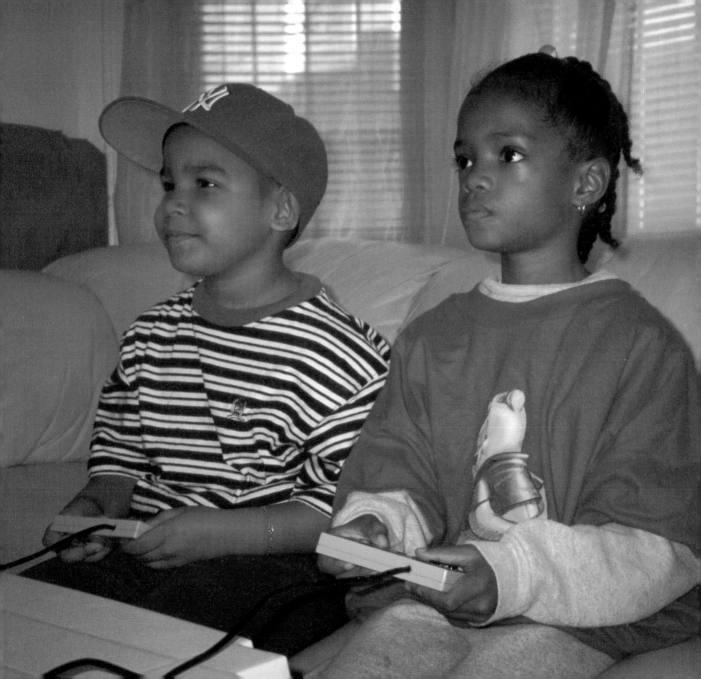

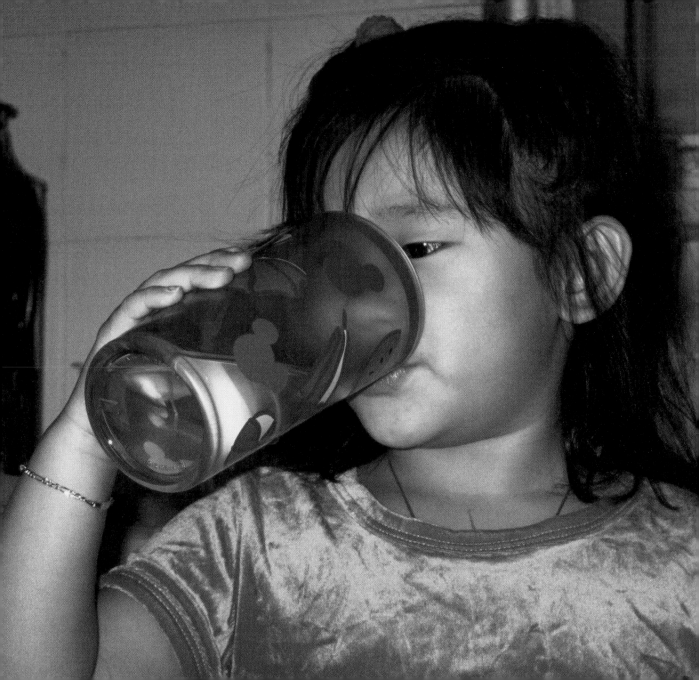

Staying Healthy and Fit

Here are some things you can do to keep your body healthy and fit:

- Play outdoors instead of watching TV.
- Snack on apples or carrots instead of cookies and candy.
- Don't eat a lot of sugar or fat.
- Be active.
- Find a sport or activity you really like, and do it often.
- Don't eat unless you are hungry.
- Stay **hydrated** by drinking lots of water.

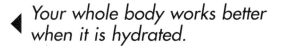

Your whole body works better when it is hydrated.

Every Body Is Different

Kids' bodies are always growing and changing. Some bodies grow faster than others. Your body may not look the same as your friends' bodies, and that's okay. You and your friends may be tall or short, thin or overweight, or a little of everything! Everyone's body is different and **unique**. The important thing is to eat well and stay active so your body will be healthy. A healthy body is a happy body!

Glossary

diet (DY-it) The food you usually eat.

efficiently (ih-FIH-shent-lee) Working in the quickest, best way possible.

energy (EH-ner-jee) A force in nature and in humans that makes activity.

exercise (EK-ser-syz) Running, swimming, biking, and other activities that use different parts of your body.

fuel (FYOOL) Something used to make energy, warmth, or power.

hydrated (HY-dray-ted) Full of water.

overweight (oh-ver-WAYT) Weighing more than is healthy for your age and height.

unique (yoo-NEEK) One of a kind.

well-balanced (WEL-BA-linst) Meals that have many different foods and nutrients in them.

Index